BE BEAUTIFUL
The Country Way

COUNTRY WAY BOOKS

Be Beautiful

THE COUNTRY WAY

Celia Haddon

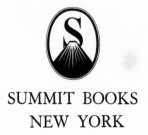

SUMMIT BOOKS
NEW YORK

Copyright © 1978 by Celia Haddon
All rights reserved
including the right of reproduction
in whole or in part in any form
Published by *Summit Books*
A Simon and Schuster Division of Gulf & Western Corporation
Simon & Schuster Building
1230 Avenue of the Americas
New York, New York 10020
Manufactured in the United States of America
Printed by The Murray Printing Company
Bound by The Book Press, Inc.
1 2 3 4 5 6 7 8 9 10

Library of Congress Cataloging in Publication Data

Haddon, Celia.
Be beautiful.

(Country way books)
Includes index.
1. Beauty, Personal. 2. Cosmetics. I. Title.
II. Series.
RA778.H16   646.7′2   78-31775

ISBN 0-671-40090-8

For Betty Mitcham

Contents

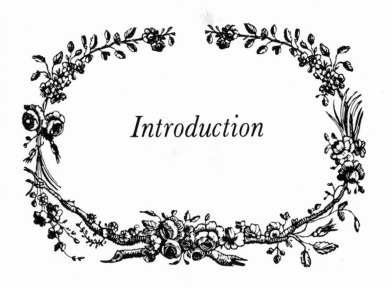

Introduction

THE MEREST GLANCE at the average dressing table will show you how efficient and far ranging are our modern shop-bought cosmetics. There are emulsifying creams, foundations, powders, lipsticks, lipgloss, eye shadow, cleansing liquids, astringents, tear-proof lash-building mascaras, deodorants, anti-perspirants, lotions and potions. There is practically no end to the methods that modern cosmetics use to promise you beauty.

And the beauty they promise comes from an extremely efficient grasp of chemicals. Face powder, alone, is high technology. Did you know that one sort of face powder contains chalk, kaolin, magnesium storeate, zinc oxide and titanium oxide? Or that one kind of hair spray is made up of a resinous substance with the incredible space fiction name of polyvinylpyrrolidone. How lucky we are. What riches of sterile, double tested, highly technological cosmetics we have offered to us. And yet . . . could we have lost something?

Consider a moment about three hundred years ago when the eccentric antiquarian John Aubrey was writing a biographical sketch of his relation Sir John Danvers. He

9

remembered walking in the garden with Sir John and wrote:

> Sir John, being my Relation and faithfull Friend, was wont in fair mornings in Summer to brush his Beaver-hatt on the Hysop and Thyme, which did perfume it with its naturall Spirit; and would last a morning or longer.

Today, of course, the modern Sir John would not bother. He would know that the quick flick of an aerosol would bring more powerful perfumes. Like pink lilac. Modern cosmetic manufacturers do not need lilac. Oh no. Pink lilac can be made up with benzyl acetate, terpineol, phenyl ethyl alcohol, heliotropin, anisic aldehyde, cinnamic alcohol, hydroxy citronellal, iso-eugenol, and phenyl acetic aldehyde, ten per cent.

The time is past, if you believe the cosmetic technology, when Bacon the essayist could write:

> Because the breath of flowers is far sweeter in the air (where it comes and goes like the warbling of music) than in the hand, therefore nothing is more fit for that delight than to know what be the flowers and plants that do best perfume the air.

Yet thousands of gardeners still plant the old plants, the violets, sweet briar, wallflowers ('which are very delightful to be set under a parlour or lower chamber window'), pinks, primroses, honeysuckles and others that he recommends. If you are, or would be, that kind of gardener then perhaps the sterilized perfumes of modern cosmetics are not enough for you.

For we are only a generation or so away from older scents—lavender bags, mothballs, *pot-pourri*, quince cheese, pomanders, cinnamon bark. A generation ago all these had their times and their seasons and each was enjoyed at its proper moment. Today modern chemists can capture, fix and infinitely reproduce the perfume of all of them.

10

But by so doing they forget that no pleasure should last forever. I think the secret of those past perfumes was their very imperfection, their impermanency. They did not last forever. Nor did the washes and the oils and the unguents, with which they were captured and made useful, react perfectly. Only natural ingredients were used, and like many of nature's finest gifts these often are only good when fresh.

Our grandmothers who bottled, and dried, and mixed knew that. They realized that the most intense pleasures are, of necessity, transient.

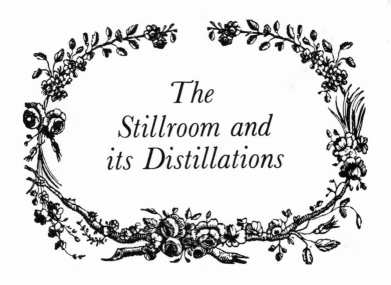

The Stillroom and its Distillations

IN AN EARLIER more innocent age every large house had its stillroom. It was not used for the production of illicit poteen from potatoes, though its principle piece of equipment was a still.

'Few families are without an alembic still' wrote Sir John Hill in 1820. He promised:

> an account of all those English plants which are remarkable for their virtues, and of the drugs that are produced by vegetables of other countries . . . also directions for the gathering and preserving roots, herbs, flowers and seeds; the various methods of preserving those simple for present use; receipts for making distilled waters, conserves, syrups, electuaries, juleps, draughts etc etc; with necessary cautions in giving them.

Most of these operations took place in the stillroom, though the kitchen with its oven might occasionally be used as well. The importance of the stillroom can be seen in the household establishment of Longleat. There were forty-three staff in all, of which twenty-eight were women. In addition to eight housemaids, two serving maids, six laundry maids and a whole range of women in the kitchen, there were two full-time stillroom maids.

At the turn of the century, the work of the stillroom maid included pickling, preserving, candying and bottling fruits and vegetables, drying herbs and flowers, and distilling sweet scented waters whose very names have a fragrance.

There were Lavender Water, Orange Flower Water and, for clearing away pimples, Pimpernel Water. But there were others, more complicated, Celestial Water, Magisterial Balm Water, Compound Balm Water, sometimes known as *Eau de Carmes*. There were also Germain Sweet-Scented Water, Sweet-Honey Water, Imperial Water, Odiferous Water, Ladies' Water, Venice Water, and even Angelic Water.

Some were merely aromatic. Others had medicinal virtues. '*Eau de Carmes* has long been famous at Paris and London . . . It has the reputation of being a cordial of very extraordinary virtues, and not only of availing in cases of the gout in the stomach' pronounced *The Toilet of Flora, or a Collection of the Most Simple and Approved Methods of preparing Baths, Essences, Pomatums, Powders, Perfumes and Sweet-Scented Waters*, published in 1784.

From the same source we learn that 'Imperial Water . . . takes away wrinkles, and renders the skin extremely delicate; it also whitens the teeth and abates the toothache, sweetens the breath and strengthens the gums. Foreign ladies prize it highly.'

Complicated recipes (called receipts in those days) were in use. Venice Water, for instance, was distilled from cow's milk, lemon slices, oranges, sugar and borax. But in the mysterious East the same cosmetic water was made differently.

This water is counterfeited at Bagdat in Persia in the following manner. Take twelve lemons peeled and sliced, twelve new-

14

laid eggs, six sheep's trotters, four ounces of sugar candy, a large slice of melon, and another of Pompion, with two drachms of Borax; distil in a large glass alembic with a leaden head.

Surely no mean feat, this! It is, of course, possible to fix up amateur stills with kettles, tubing and other equipment. But it is difficult and arguably dangerous. But we can imitate our ancestors. Hungary Water was perhaps the best-known distilled water and was used to recruit strength and dispel gloominess. It retained its popularity until recently. Using simple ingredients obtainable at most good chemists or grocers we can still make Hungary Water – or, at least, an enjoyable imitation.

To make your own Hungary Water simply mix rosewater and witch hazel, with a proportion of rosewater double that of witch hazel. The rosewater provides the scent and sweetness. The witch hazel is a fairly fierce astringent. Hungary Water can be used as a facial astringent, but is perhaps rather fierce for dry or tender skins. A little vodka will dilute it further and, if you wish, you can leave herbs in the mixture overnight to elaborate the fragrance – though bear in mind that they may also add colour. Vodka tends to turn brown with rosemary, while pink rose petals change the usually colourless rosewater to a yellowy-pink.

Many modern herbals give recipes for making perfumed rubbing lotions, using either rectified spirits or rubbing alcohol. I have asked for these at chemists and have been told they cannot be sold over the counter, so I am unable to know how well they would absorb the fragrance of either herbs or flowers left in them to soak. Those who have friends working in laboratories may be able to beg some laboratory alcohol to experiment.

Surgical spirit seems to be the only substitute on open sale. The only surgical spirit I have been able to buy has a somewhat unpleasant odour, added, I imagine, to stop people drinking it as a cheap substitute for vodka. Soaking herbs and flowers in surgical spirit is therefore not entirely

15

rewarding. It does not smell like those old sweet distilled waters. But a strong herb like rosemary or mint will add something to the original smell.

Using a pestle and mortar, bruise the herb well. You will need enough herbs to fill a quarter of a bottle and then add sufficient spirit to fill the bottle. Leave the bottle in the sunlight or in a warm place for two weeks. Then strain and rebottle. Repeat the process of soaking fresh herbs in the liquid, if you want a stronger-smelling lotion. You will have quite a reasonable alcohol lotion to rub on the body – refreshing, for instance, if used on tired feet.

The other alternative is to damn the expense and turn to vodka. It is colourless and without any strong smell, except for those delicious Polish varieties with grasses in them. The same principle of bruising the herb, and leaving it to stand in a bottle of vodka in sunlight applies.

I imagine this could well be a culinary rather than a cosmetic product, as long as the herb is not left too long. I am told, though I have not tried it, that lemon peel in vodka gives a delicious flavour. But my advice is to experiment first with only a little of the liquid, since it is expensive. If you like what develops, then expand production.

Vinegar is the other liquid which can be used as a base for our stillroom substitutes. In our ancestors' time herbal vinegars were more than just a treat for the salad bowl. They were an important adjunct to health. Cardinal Wolsey, it is said, always carried with him a flask of Marseilles Vinegar, also known as Four Thieves Vinegar, to ward off the plague. 'To a gallon of white wine vinegar add rosemary tops, sage flowers, lavender, rue, camphor and cloves' is the recipe from *The Practice of Perfumery*, subtitled *A Treatise on the Toilet and Cosmetic Arts, Historical, Scientific and Practical*, published in the last century.

Herbal vinegars can be made with any of the common herbs – thyme, mint, rosemary and so forth. Tarragon vinegar is perhaps the best for eating. As a rubbing lotion or as a refreshment to the spirits on a handkerchief try lavender vinegar or even rose petal vinegar. Some writers suggest violet vinegars, but I cannot bring myself to pluck their flowers so ruthlessly, even if the herbalist Culpeper was right when he said that a poultice of the leaves and flowers made with water or wine 'eases pains in the head, caused through want of sleep.' Floral and herbal vinegars make pretty gifts, if a sprig of the plant is left in the bottle. But do choose good quality wine vinegar. Otherwise the herbal fragrance will be overpowered.

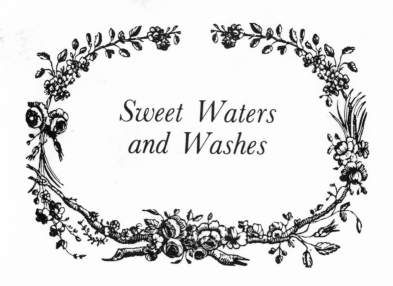

Sweet Waters and Washes

'DABBLING IN THE DEW makes the milkmaid fair' was the refrain of a romantic ballad that my mother used to sing at the piano with *her* mother. She taught it to me, and told me that old piece of folklore about the dew on midsummer morning: 'If you walk barefoot through the dew that morning, you will become beautiful.'

Does it work? It certainly is a pleasure, and there is a long tradition behind it. For years women have used dew or rainwater to wash with. Even in the humblest cottager's home, the woman of the family used rainwater from the barrel rather than well water for her toilet. 'Rain-water was supposed to be good for the complexion' writes Flora Thompson in *Lark Rise to Candleford*, an enchanting book about Oxford village life at the end of the last century. The women she wrote about had little or no money but 'though they had no money to spend upon beautifying themselves, they were not too far gone in poverty to neglect such means as they had to that end.'

Though we may not be able to distil sweet water like our more wealthy ancestors, we can benefit from the more simple remedies of the poor. Anybody can make their own rosewater – not the distilled kind. Just boil rose petals in water for a few minutes and use the liquid as a sweet wash for the face.

Other simple home cosmetics were by-products of the kitchen. The water in which spinach had been boiled was saved for a cleansing facial wash, so too was the water in which fresh beans had been cooked. (Vegetable matter tends to extract rather than put in moisture to the face, so these are best used for people with oily rather than dry skins.)

The most famous face lotion of all came from the summer hedgerows. Elderflowers were gathered and distilled in the

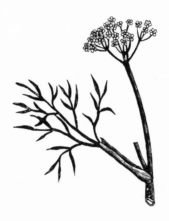

stillrooms of the rich. Culpeper points out that it 'is of much use to clean the skin from sun-burning, freckles, morphew or the like; and takes away the head-ache, coming of a cold cause, the head being bathed therein.'

In the cottages, away from the big house, elderflowers were used more simply. Boiled in rainwater or in spring water and used to wash the face, they acted as a simple astringent. Add a little glycerine, or a small amount of alcohol (vodka will do) and the mixture is particularly good. Naturally, it will not keep forever, though placing it in the refrigerator will extend its life.

In *The Cook's and Confectioner's Dictionary, or the Accomplish'd Housewife's Companion* of 1723 I have discovered a recipe for clove water. 'Mix a little Cinnamon with the Cloves, or else the Scent is apt to be too Strong' writes John Nott, cook to the Duke of Bolton. 'Allow half a score of Cloves to a Quart of Water, put in a good Piece of Sugar; let them infuse for some time over hot Embers, or in a warm place; then strain it for use.' I imagine this clove water is for drinking or cookery, because of the addition of sugar. But without the sugar, it makes a pleasing washing lotion, either for the face or perhaps to be added to the bath.

Much simpler is the recipe for facial beauty of Baroness Staffe, a French aristocrat whose beauty book was translated by an equally aristocratic Englishwoman, Lady Colin Campbell. She considered a walk in the rain one of the best facial cosmetics available. To cleanse the skin thoroughly she suggested another absolutely free remedy. Just wet a towel or a cloth in boiling water, then wring it out. Place this over the face, reclining at ease for half an hour – preferably (I think) while listening to music or the radio.

The Baroness also argued that too much heat dried the skin – something that is true today in centrally heated houses. Doctors who deal with elderly people confirm the Baroness's experience. Air conditioning also removes the moisture from the air. The modern expensive remedy is to buy a humidifier. The Baroness's absolutely free tip was simply to make sure there are bowls or jars of water in all heated rooms. They can, after all, have flowers in them – or even be full of water in which herbs or flowers have been boiled, as long as this is changed when necessary.

Milk is the other natural cleansing lotion. Milkmaids did not have to rely on the dew. They could wash their face straight from the cow. Milk and brandy mixed, and dabbed on the face *after* washing, is said to tone up the skin. One of the wise ideas of our great-grandmothers was that sunburn was bad for the skin. Today dermatologists will tell you that there was a lot in those old ideas. Sunburn is the skin's protection against the sun, and there is absolutely no doubt that sun produces wrinkles. The most wrinkled men and women are fair-skinned nudists, it is always said. Our milkmaid used buttermilk against sunburn. 'A young lady-farmer of my acquaintance' wrote the Baroness, with a surprising lapse into democracy, 'never uses anything but sour buttermilk.'

A more exotic recipe, using fresh cream is to be found in another Victorian book *The Practice of Perfumery*. It consists of an ounce of cream, eight ounces of milk, one ounce of *eau de Cologne*, an ounce of lemon and a drachm of sugar. With a confidence in powerful-sounding chemicals, which I am far from sharing, it also suggests adding alum. After shaking all this together, you applied it to freckles which then magically disappeared. I think one would be better keeping one's freckles.

Finally, wine was often used for washing – white wines for fair skins and red wine for oily or dark skins. Again, it seems quite powerfully astringent to me, but there is the advantage of being able to drink it either before, after, or during the beauty treatment.

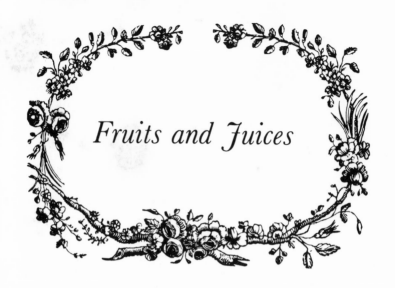

Fruits and Juices

JUST AS ONE MAY PLEASE both skin and stomach with wine, so the fruits of summer have cosmetic as well as culinary pleasures. Strawberry juice is an old remedy. Liquidize the fruit, wipe it over the face and, as long as your greed for strawberries outweighs worries about dirt on the face, eat it. At this moment I have to confess that I am so passionately fond of strawberries that I think this is rather a waste of their fruit. But I rely on that old herbalist John Gerard who suggests that even taken internally, they may still be a cosmetic. 'The ripe Strawberries quench thirst, and take away, if they be often used, the rednesse and heat of the face.' He also says 'The distilled water drunke with white Wine is good against the passion of the heart, reviving the spirits, and making the heart merry.'

Raspberries are another favourite. Culpeper writes:

Venus owns this shrub. The fruit . . . has a pleasant grateful smell and taste, is cordial and strengthens the stomach, stays vomiting, is somewhat astringent, and good to prevent miscarriage. The fruit is very grateful as nature presents it, but made into a sweetmeat with sugar or fermented with Wine, the flavour is improved. It is fragrant, a little acide, and of a cooling nature. It dissolves the tartarous concretions on the teeth, but is inferior to strawberries for that purpose. . . .

Raspberries and strawberries for cleaning off the tartar are a delicious thought. If only my dentist would prescribe them for me. (It is perhaps worth pointing out that, fruit apart, there is no *need* for toothpaste, except in so far as its

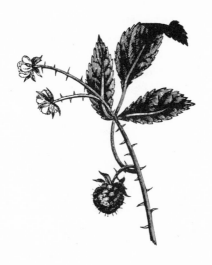

fluoride content is useful for growing children. Brushing the teeth without toothpaste is just as effective.)

A generation or two ago, the strawberry and raspberry season must have been greeted with relief as well as pleasure. For the recipes given in old Victorian beauty books have frightening chemical contents – cuttle fish powder, cream of tartar, and orris-root powder is one of the kindest from *The Girl's Own Paper* of 1894.

For an even earlier generation gunpowder was often recommended.

This will remove every spot and blemish, and give your Teeth an inconceivable whiteness. It is almost needless to say, that the mouth must be well washed after this operation, for besides the necessity of so doing, the saltpetre etc. used in the composition of the Gunpowder, would, if it remained, prove injurious to the Gums.

Next after strawberry juice, as a fruity cosmetic with many uses, must come the lemon. Lemon juice is often recommended for cleaning the face in the old beauty books, but only those people with oily skins should use it undiluted. A kinder lotion can be made up with a wineglassful of the juice, a pint of rainwater, and five drops of rosewater. This will freshen the skin. When you have pressed out the lemon juice, do not throw away the lemon peel as this will remove tar stains from the hands or arms. Another old wives' recommendation is to take the two halves of the fruit (after

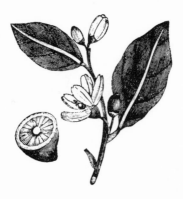

squeezing the juice) and rest your elbows inside them to whiten the skin. Some people also use lemons to clean the skin around the nails, by pushing each finger inside the cut half of a lemon and turning it round and round. But for nail-biters like myself I think it would probably be too painful.

The cucumber is another traditional country cosmetic. Slice it and lay the pieces over the eyes and forehead to freshen and relieve nervous tension. (Having to lie still for a minute or so while doing this also calms the nerves.) Cucumber is an astringent, and if its skin is removed and the flesh liquidized the pulp can be used on the face in the same way as strawberries. A melon, it is said by some, has similar properties, but it seems to me they are too exotic a fruit to use in this fashion.

Those who have plenty of time and money may like to try Baroness Staffe's lavish recipe for cucumber cream. The quantities are her own, and to my mind are really far too much. But no doubt they could be cut down in proportion. Another major problem is the time it requires, all right no doubt in the days of stillroom maids but certainly far too long for me. She started with a peeled cucumber and a peeled melon. Both were cut into small pieces after the seeds had been removed. To these pieces were added one pound of clarified lard and half a pint of fresh milk, and the whole concoction was simmered in a *bain marie* for ten hours without letting it come to the boil. The mixture was left to congeal and then washed several times in cold running water until the water ran clear. It was then put in pots. Somehow I do not think I shall ever do this, myself, but it is an interesting reminder of the time and energy our great grandmothers had.

Apples provide another early cosmetic recipe, this time for hand cream.

Beat some peeled Apples (having first taken out the cores) in a marble mortar, with Rose Water and White Wine, of each equal parts. Add some Crumb of Bread, blanched Almonds, and a little White Soap; and simmer the whole over a slow fire till it acquires a proper consistence.

The tomato was a fruit which the early herbalists regarded with some suspicion. Gerard knew tomatoes as 'apples of love'.

In Spaine and those hot Regions they use to eate the Apples prepared and boiled with pepper, salt and oyle; but they yeeld very little nourishment to the body, and the same naught and corrupt.

By the nineteenth century, tomatoes were gaining acceptance. 'The plant is a kind of nightshade' wrote Sir John Hill. 'We cultivate it in gardens. The Italians eat the fruits as we do cucumbers. The juice is cooling and is good, used externally in eruptions on the skin.' By the time Mrs Beeton had started her writing, she recommended rubbing sliced ripe tomatoes on the arms to whiten them. Massage the juice into the skin and leave it to dry. Then wash the arms and, finally, rub in some cold cream. It seems rather elaborate for white arms.

At this point I cannot resist giving the most charming cure for hiccups I have ever encountered. It probably does not work. It certainly is not a cosmetic. But it is irresistable. 'For the Hickup' wrote E. Smith in the 1744 edition of *The Compleat Houfewife or Accomplifh'd Gentlewoman's Companion.* 'Take three or four preserv'd damsons in your mouth at a time and swallow them by degrees.'

It would spoil everything, if this was done with prunes!

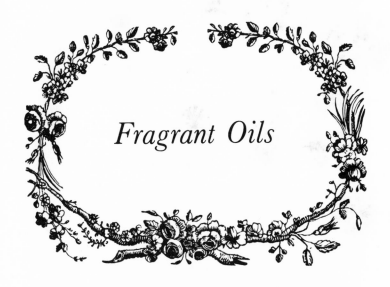

Fragrant Oils

'THE VEGETABLE KINGDOM is indeed the El Dorado of the perfumer – tree, shrub, herb, and flower vieing with each other in sweet rivalry in the richness and delicacy of their perfume' wrote a Victorian perfume expert.

Nearly all the highly perfumed flowers and leaves have their own essential oils. Some technical books suggest pressing huge quantities of these to collect the resulting oil. Or by distilling, it is apparently sometimes possible to collect an oil that appears on the surface of the distilled water. But both these methods are quite out of the question for the ordinary individual. We need go no further than Culpeper to learn the answer. In the seventeenth century we have a perfectly good recipe for a fragrant oil – ie, one made up of herbs and oil combined.

> The way of making them is this; having bruised the herbs or flowers you make your oil of, put them into an earthen pot, and to two or three handfuls of them pour a pint of oil, cover the pot with a paper, set it in the sun about a fortnight or so, according as the sun is in hotness: then having warmed it very well by the

fire, press out the herb, etc very hard in a press, and add as many more herbs to the same oil – bruise the herbs (I mean not the oil) in like manner, set them in the sun as before; the oftener you repeat this, the stronger your oil will be; at last, when you conceive it strong enough, boil both oil and herbs together, till the juice be consumed, which you may know by its leaving its bubbling, and the herbs will be crisp; then strain it while it is hot, and keep it in a stone or glass vessel for your use.

The general use of these oils is for pains in the limbs, roughness in the skin, the itch, etc as also for ointments and plaisters.

These oils are also vital ingredients for some of the cosmetic creams described later in this book. You can, if you wish, purchase fragrant oils over the counter – spike lavender oil is one of them. But the fun of making your own natural beauty aids includes, I think, the use of one's home-made fragrant oils.

To Culpeper's recipe little more need be added, except that today it seems better to keep the original herb and oil mixture in a glass jar or bottle. Some writers recommend adding a spoonful of vinegar or vodka. When I have done this the oil has gone slightly cloudy so I think oil alone is better. The herbs you can use are really endless – marjoram, thyme, lovage, bergamot, mints of all kinds, tansy, or even bitter rue, if you enjoy its weird fragrance. Or you can mix them together to make mingled fragrances. Flowers are also a possibility, and I see no reason why one might not experiment with the contents of the spice cupboard and try cloves, cardamom or coriander.

The biggest poser is which oil to use as the base. People have their own preferences and I can only suggest careful sniffs at more than a few bottles. Most writers agree that ordinary cooking oil is unsuitable but there remains corn oil, safflower oil, olive oil and even linseed oil quite apart from the expensive almond oil.

For the treatment of sprains and bruises I rather favour linseed oil. It is a heavy very smelly oil that some people dislike. Because I was brought up on a farm, I have the fondest memory of linseed. It used to be used in hot bran mashes for tired horses, and as the steaming mixture was taken into the loose boxes, I can remember thinking how delicious it smelt. With linseed oil, you will need a strong herb like rosemary and even so the linseed smell will still be there.

For cosmetics a lighter oil is necessary. Corn oil is suggested, but despite its harvesty smell I don't find I enjoy it very much. I am far more fond of olive oil. Olive oil, without additional perfume, rubbed on the skin makes me think of hot Mediterranean beaches and delicious salads.

With olive oil one can make, for instance, *Huile Antique de la Rose*. An old recipe suggests a pound of olive oil and a pound of fresh rose petals. 'Infuse for seven days with relays of fresh flowers, straining off the oil each time.' If you do not have enough rose petals try honeysuckle. (But do not take the petals from the hedgerows. Grow your own.) Its French name is *Huile Antique au Chèvre Feuille*.

Lavender oil, made by infusing flowers in olive oil, is another summer pleasure – if you have enough lavender bushes. As I have to choose between lavender oil and lavender bags (not having enough for both) I am afraid I do not make the oil.

If you do not like olive oil safflower is probably the best alternative. It does not smell very much and takes the fragrance from the herb without too much undertone of its own flavour.

Some books recommend using primroses and cowslips in oil. Our grandmothers made cowslip wine and cowslip balls and cowslip tea without a second thought. But today, when such flowers are becoming scarce, I do not think it is justified. I *do* have primroses in my garden but even so I cannot bear to pick them. And as for plucking my double mauve primroses . . . perish the thought.

Perhaps the best oil of all for cosmetics is almond oil. It can be bought from a good chemist, but it is expensive, and unfortunately this whole system of soaking flowers and herbs in oil inevitably means wasting some of the oil. I recommend testing out a herbal fragrance on a cheaper oil, before using almond oil.

There is also that liquid so dreaded in the nursery of the past – liquid paraffin. If you suffer from dry skin too much soap and water can be harmful. The cheapest way of washing the face with an odourless compound is to use liquid paraffin. I have tried infusing herbs in liquid paraffin with interesting results. To speed up the infusions with other oils I try to shake the container well once a day. With liquid

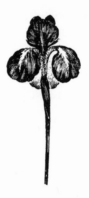

paraffin this is not so simple as it is much thicker than the oils and the herbs tend to stay at the bottom, only moving (and slowly) if you turn the whole vessel upside down. But they *do* infuse, colouring the otherwise colourless liquid and giving it some of their odour. It is certainly worth doing, if you need to have a cheap non-oily face lotion. It is also useful as a base for other herbal cosmetics. But the infusion is neither quite so fast nor so effective as with the oils.

A quicker way to get a herbal oil is simply to use it as a sort of fry-up. Sir John Hill recommends boiling one pound of elder flowers in a quart of olive oil till the flowers are crisp, in order to obtain elder oil. Using the same method he obtains what he calls 'green oil'. The herbal ingredients are three ounces of camomile, three ounces of bay leaves, sea-wormwood, rue and sweet marjoram. These oils are to rub into pained or swollen limbs.

Another oil is orris root oil. The orris is an iris which grows in the garden, unremarked for its perfume. It is, in fact, one of those plants that Francis Bacon classified as 'fast flowers of their smells; so that you may walk by a whole row of them and find nothing of their sweetness; yea though it be in a morning's dew.' The perfume of this iris comes, in fact, from its root not its flowers. Dried and powdered, they smell of violet and have a reputation for keeping their scent well. So far, I have bought mine ready powdered, but am planning to try and grow my own. The root needs to be cut into small slivers and then baked in the oven.

Nearly all these oils have more than one use. Many of them, particularly the ones made with olive oil, can be eaten in salads or used in cookery. Others are just a haunting, if transient perfume, when rubbed on the body. But you will need a stock of them if you are going to take the next step of making your own country unguents.

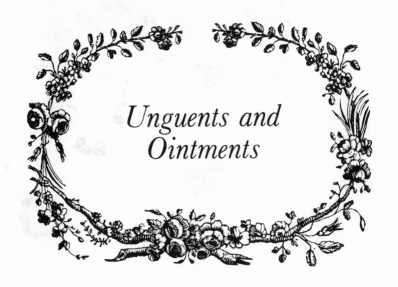

Unguents and Ointments

'PIGS FOR HEALTH' was an old Victorian saying, and for the typical country cottager in those days a pig was not only a source of health but of beauty too. Bacon was the main meat ingredient of their diet, and in a family economy where spare cash was almost non-existent the pig provided a base for many kinds of ointments and creams. Olive or other oils were simply out of reach of the housewife's purse. *The Family Herbal* of Sir John Hill is clear on this. One of its basic ointments was simply melted lard with the relevant herbs, bruised and chopped, added to the fat. The fat was heated till the herbs were crisp then strained. For a stronger infusion a second helping of herbs was fried up. The result is a hard green ointment. There is no denying that even with modern clarified cooking lards, there remains a lingering aroma of pig. As a pig-lover, I have happily used this green ointment as a kind of barrier cream on my hands before gardening, and as a hand cream after washing up. The herb continues to smell, and I don't really mind the pig aroma.

Clarified mutton fat was also used in the same way. (Being

less fond of sheep I have not tried this.) Goose fat was also highly esteemed as a remedy to be rubbed on bronchial chests, and as a soothing ointment for chilblains. Today I am chilblain free, and in my chilblainy childhood I did not know a goose so I cannot judge its efficacy. But the advantage of Sir John Hill's green lard, clarified mutton fat, or herbal goose grease is that all three will make a gourmet cooking medium if you do not like the result as a cosmetic.

These fatty concoctions, however, are primitive. The transition towards proper creams and ointments involves two vital ingredients, beeswax and emulsifying wax. Obtaining them is not easy. Your best hope is to speak nicely to your local chemist and ask him to order them. (A London supplier is listed at the end of this book.)

The beeswax stiffens the oil or fat which is your easiest basic ingredient. The emulsifying wax enables you to add liquids like rosewater to the mixture. In the past spermaceti was used for this, and some unthinking cosmetic firms unfortunately still use it. But spermaceti comes from whales, highly intelligent warm-blooded creatures which are threatened with over-fishing by the whaling fleets. (Did you know that the oceans of the world are full of long drawn-out songs, which the animals sing to each other over hundreds of miles?) Killing whales to make cosmetics is unjustifiable.

The principle of making ointments is to vary the proportion of beeswax to oil. The more beeswax the harder the ointment will be. Personally I use oil rather than fat, because having bought the beeswax it seems foolish to save a few pence simply by using lard instead of oil. A basic proportion for a creamy consistency is eight parts of oil to one part of beeswax, but first experiment with small quantities as the results vary with different ingredients.

The other alternatives to oil are petroleum jelly or liquid paraffin. Both of these seem to me to make a slightly lighter ointment, more liquid, that is. Some books say that you can use lanolin but the only brand I have been able to obtain did not mix with the beeswax.

If you have already infused your oil or liquid paraffin with herbal fragrances, they will probably be a rather pleasant greenish colour. (It has been suggested to me that petroleum jelly can be made to smell of herbs by bruising the herbs using a pestle and mortar, adding them to the jelly, and leaving them for a day or two.) You will need a *bain marie*, or double boiler for the next stage. (One small saucepan balanced in a larger one with boiling water in it, or a pudding basin placed inside a saucepan of boiling water will do instead.) Just melt the beeswax in the oil, liquid paraffin or petroleum jelly.

You can make a very effective lipsalve by just using beeswax and olive oil in a proportion of about 1:6 respectively. (Less olive oil if you want a firmer salve. You can always reheat and change the proportion if the first try does not work.) Pour this when still liquid into an old cleaned-out lipstick container and harden it in the refrigerator.

The recipe for cold cream is more complicated. It is said that the Greek physician Galen invented this. His recipe was simply six ounces of white beeswax heated with a pound of oil of roses, into which was stirred a cupful of water. It does not work. I have tried substituting oil and liquid paraffin for the rose oil (as some herbal books suggest) but the water just doesn't mix in. The missing ingredient is the emulsifying wax. If you add roughly the same amount of emulsifying wax, as beeswax, then the water (with a dash of spirit) will mix in, foaming slightly in the saucepan. (Prolonged keeping of this in a warm room may mean that the oil and water will eventually separate out again.)

A friend of mind, Rosie Atkins, has made a very effective cleansing cream. Rosie's cream is made with half an ounce of beeswax, half an ounce of emulsifying wax, four ounces of petroleum jelly, one ounce of witch hazel and three ounces of rosewater. You melt the wax, emulsifying wax and petroleum jelly in the double boiler, stirring hard, and gradually add the other liquids.

These are large quantities, because Rosie gives away pots

of her cream to friends. But if you keep the basic proportions in mind you can simply halve or even quarter the recipe. In fact, exact measurements do not seem to matter too much as long as one does not add too much petroleum jelly or oil, or try to get too much water incorporated. Exactly the same recipe can be adapted to make different cold creams, as long as the beeswax and emulsifying wax remain. You can add vodka and water instead of witch hazel and rosewater. You can also use liquid paraffin or oil instead of petroleum jelly. Part of the fun is experimenting.

Having made your own unguents and ointments, use them.

An old country remedy for sore, chapped or overworked hands is sleeping in gloves impregnated with fat or oil. For badly dirtied hands another recipe is to rub on a mixture of olive oil and salt before washing it off with soap. It leaves the

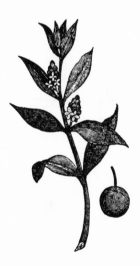

skin feeling exceptionally clean. If you find making your own cold cream rather difficult (and I have had one or two failures, myself) console yourself with the thought of what earlier housewives had to do. In the *Toilet of Flora*, there is an amazingly elaborate, not to say costly, recipe for hand cream.

> A Paste for the Hands . . . Take Sweet Almond, half a pound; White Wine Vinegar, Brandy and Spring Water, of each two quarts, two ounces of Crumb of Bread, and the Yolks of two Eggs. Blanch and beat the Almonds, moistening them with the Vinegar; add the Crumb of Bread soaked in the Brandy and mix it with the Almonds and Yolks of Egg, by repeated Tirturation. Then pour in the Water, and simmer the whole over a slow fire, keeping the composition continually stirring, till it has acquired a proper consistence.

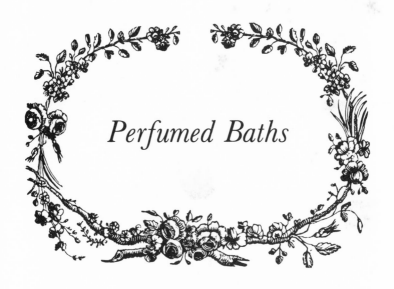

Perfumed Baths

WOULD YOU BE SURPRISED to know that a long hot bath
is positively medicinal? 'In cases of internal inflammation
and congestion and of bilious colic, there is no more certain
remedy than a hot bath. It is also known to have worked
surprising cures in cases of obstinate constipation' wrote the
Baroness Staffe. The link between baths and constipation
would no doubt prove fruitful for Freudian analysts. On
safer ground, one can point out that there has always been a
link between bathing and beauty.

In ancient times baths were magnificent occasions. Nero's
wife Poppaea bathed in asses' milk, in strawberry juice, and
in a bath made of porphyry. (Whether the asses' milk was
mixed with strawberry juice, or the two taken separately I
do not know.) In sixteenth-century France Diane de
Poitiers, mistress of the King, bathed daily in rainwater – an
eccentric habit at a time when baths were the exception
rather the rule. By the eighteenth century, however,
exotic baths were almost commonplace among the rich.
Milk of almonds was highly recommended, as were melon
juice, green barley water, linseed water and even weak veal

broth. (If one lingered long enough in the latter, might it have congealed into a sort of jellied consommé, one wonders?)

The cheapest way of enjoying an exotic bath today is to add the natural flowers and leaves from the garden. All kinds of flowers have been recommended and no doubt all kinds can be enjoyed. But I hope we can leave violets,

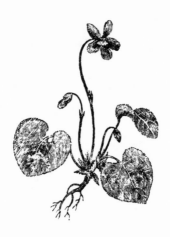

primroses and cowslips to bloom in the hedgerows and fields where they look so beautiful. Rose petals in the bath look pretty and smell prettier. But mine are usually being dried for various schemes, so there never seem to be enough. Marigold petals are good too.

But the baths I have most enjoyed are those that include sprays of either lovage or mint. (Together they do not seem quite so pleasant.) Lovage is a wonderful herb with beautiful strong green leaves and a faint smell of celery though I would not go so far as Culpeper who maintained that it resisted poison. Mints are a great pleasure. Many people just associate mint with the run-of-the-mill plant found being rather a nuisance in the vegetable patch (though good for new potatoes). In fact there are several different flavours of mint, of which I like apple mint and orange mint (also known as *Eau de Cologne* mint) much better than spearmint, the most common variety.

Those who do not feel at ease lying in a bath surrounded by sprays of greenstuff could make little muslin bags in which to put the fresh herb, but I think this is a terrible waste of effort. If you must keep the leaves away from your sight, just stuff them into bags made by cutting the legs from old nylon stockings or tights and knotting them at each end. It does not look very pretty, but at least it avoids the labour of sewing.

The Toilet of Flora suggests preparing aromatic water before the bath begins.

Boil, for the space of two or three minutes, in a sufficient quantity of river water, one or more of the following plants; viz Laurel, Thyme, Rosemary, Wild Thyme, Sweet-Marjoram, Bastard-Marjoram, Lavender, Southernwood, Wormwood,

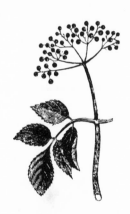

Sage, Pennyroyal, Sweet Basil, Balm, Wild Mint, Hyssop, Clove-july flowers, Anise, Fennel, or any other herbs that have an agreeable scent. Having strained off the liquor from the herbs, add to it a little Brandy, or camphorated Spirits of Wine.

This is an excellent Bath to strengthen the limbs; it removes pains proceeding from cold, and promotes perspiration.

39

I have no quarrel with this recipe, even if it does mean a little more effort before running the bath. There was a Victorian custom that was rather similar. For the better entertainment of guests, their bedchambers would include not only the basin and large ewer of water to wash in, but also a much smaller jug. In this small jug was a pink weakly scented water, in which rose petals had been boiled.

Of course ingredients other than herbs and flowers can be added to the bath. *The Toilet of Flora* has a recipe for a cosmetic bath that reads rather like the instructions for making a mash for horses.

> Take two pounds of Barley or Bean-meal, eight pounds of Bran, and a few handfuls of Borage Leaves. Boil these ingredients in a sufficient quantity of spring water. Nothing cleanses and softens the skin like this bath.

The cottager's equivalent bath was much more simple – just bran or oatmeal in a small muslin bag. (Today a piece of knotted stocking will do equally as well.) Fill this with about two or three handfuls of medium oatmeal, of the sort found in health shops, and use it to rub the skin while you are in the bath. It gives out a lovely milkiness, and the bag can be used three or four times. (The wild birds can eat the oatmeal that remains.) A bag filled with bran needs a little soaking in a jug or bowl for an hour or so before the bath. Use the liquid in which it has soaked for the bath, incidentally. The bath smells of harvest time and the warm fragrance of a successful autumn.

If you have made an aromatic vinegar, or rubbing alcohol, nothing is easier than to put a drop or two into the bath just before getting in. The perfume will not remain like bought smells do, but for those first few minutes it is lovely.

Exactly the same can be done with aromatic oils. As we grow older, our skins grow naturally dryer, and baths should probably be less frequent. If you wish to keep your baths, try adding some oil to them or rubbing some on the body afterwards. It need not be expensive manufactured oil. Your own aromatic oil will do.

In an earlier age when people had to walk farther, and when all hot water had to be laboriously heated up above the kitchen fire, foot baths were more common than they are now. 'Boil in water a pound of Bran, with a few Marshmallow Roots, and two or three handfuls of Mallow Leaves.' This makes 'An Emolient Bath for the Feet.'

Here is another. 'Take four handfuls of Pennyroyal, Sage and Rosemary, three handfuls of Angelica, and four ounces of Juniper Berries; boil these ingredients in a sufficient quantity of water, and strain off the liquor for use.'

Another bathtime delight is to make your own soap. Well perhaps not exactly make it from scratch. But if you have any little old odds and ends of soap around you can boil them up with a teaspoonful or more of water, then pour them into little moulds. It is easier, if the soap is not too wet, to pass it through the cheese grater first.

Then comes the fun. Add your own oatmeal or bran in equal proportion, or less, to the soap. On the whole I think a finer brand of oatmeal is best for this, but if you use too much it will not be very soapy. However, if you have a fairly dry mixture once the oatmeal has been added, you can shape your own soapcake, then roll it in oatmeal which clings to its outside. Some herbalists recommend doing the same thing with herbs or with adding distilled water. I do not see much point in this. Most soap, even the cheapest, already has its own fragrance and the added herbs would only compete. The only scentless soap I know is far from cheap.

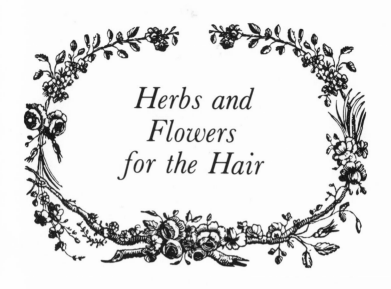

Herbs and Flowers for the Hair

WHEN I WAS A SMALL CHILD I used to stay with my grandmother on my father's side. I don't remember very much about the visits. But one occasion has stayed in my mind with surprising vividness.

It was night time in her bedroom. Heavy curtains stretching down to the floor were drawn. Her bed was one of those very large high ones, which to a child seem as if they need climbing up to as well as into. She was sitting at her dressing table and brushing her hair. It was the hair that was so remarkable. In the day-time it never seemed anything but short (in a bun perhaps?) Now it came flowing down from her head, grey in parts, white in others. She was brushing it slowly and methodically. It had never occurred to me that an old woman could have long hair.

That hair and the hair of many of her generation who had been born in the palmy days of Victoria was part of an elaborate beauty ritual. 'Brush your hair with a hundred strokes' people like Nannies used to advise. With today's short hair, that really is not necessary, but when a woman's crowning glory was that tumbling mass down to and past her shoulders a hundred strokes was necessary. But there was an art to it. It was not just brushing. The hair had to be divided into separate tresses. Each tress was then brushed thoroughly to remove all the tangles. For if the hair was brushed without this tress by tress division, tangles would remain underneath the shining surface.

There were other womanly mysteries about hair. To make hair grow longer, those in the know cut an inch off it. But not just at anytime. The cutting must be done at the new moon. Then, and only then, the cutting would stimulate its growth.

Other more common sense advice was given to those whose hair was thinning (and thinning hair is too often a by-product of old age). Change the style, the old wives would say. And if changing the style did not reduce the thinning, it probably at least concealed its extent.

Remedies against greying abounded then as they do now. 'Those who find their hair turning white would go to the Prince of Darkness himself to conceal the snows of time, and one soon perceives they have used infernal measures' wrote Baroness Staffe darkly. 'This is a sad want of commonsense. We must remain what we are, or what we have become.' Today the same infernal measures are still in use. Some of the hair dyes still legal in the British Isles include fierce chemicals. Every head has first to be tested (or ought to be) for allergy to these dyes. And there is some controversy about whether some of the chemicals produce cancer in animals.

Our grandmothers avoided these dangers when they stuck to harmless vegetable dyes. A common concoction was a rinse using proportions of half of cold tea to half of water in which sage leaves had been boiled. This was meant to darken hair, and give back colour to grey hair. (As a blonde, I have never tried this.) A less satisfactory dye was made of walnut leaves. As we all know walnut husks stain, and the disadvantage of this dye was that it stained not only the hair but also the scalp underneath. ('Oil of Walnuts frequently

43

rubbed on a child's forehead will prevent the hair from growing on that part' – a piece of eccentric information offered by *The Toilet of Flora*.)

For those with fair hair, a wash of camomile is the traditional treatment. Sometimes this is wrongly described as a hair lightener. It is not. What it does is add a yellow colour to the hair. To make the wash you simply boil camomile flowers in water for twenty minutes and use the liquid as a rinse. A strong solution may actually turn blonde hair almost chestnut. There is one flaw that applies to camomile, and I should think to sage and tea. It adds colour to the hair all right, but it also adds colour to the towel too. (It comes out in the wash.)

A more effective treatment for lightening blonde hair is a cupful of vinegar mixed with water, half and half. Some suggest cider vinegar but I prefer the aroma of white wine vinegar. If rosemary has been steeped in it, so much the better. Rosemary has a reputation of adding lustre to the hair. It certainly adds a pleasant scent. Lemon juice can be substituted for vinegar. It has a bleaching effect, but pints and pints of pure lemon juice might be rather hard on the hair. The juice of one lemon seems quite adequate.

The other natural hair aid is the egg. Egg shampoos abound on the market, but there is really no need to pay fancy prices for them. You can use either the yolk or the white or both. Either mix it into the shampoo, or use it afterwards. But whatever you do, rinse it out thoroughly with cool water. I once spent half a morning with a bit of scrambled egg white clinging to the back of my head! It seems to add body to my hair. Beer does the same. A school-friend of mine reminded me the other day of how she was almost expelled from our girls' boarding school for going into a pub. All she had wanted (though they didn't believe her) was a little beer for her hair.

A very simple recipe is given in *The Lady's Dressing Table* which may help those who have run out of shampoo. It suggests a teacupful of salt mixed with a quart of rainwater, and stood for twelve hours. Before using it, add one more cupful of hot rainwater.

A dry shampoo is the other emergency aid for the hair. If you are really pushed for time, you can make a dry shampoo just from ordinary flour. If you are lucky enough to have powdered orris root on the premises add a pinch or two of that. This is not an ideal dry shampoo but it is better than nothing, so long as you brush it out vigorously and painstakingly.

In the old beauty books hair tonics abound. Most of them promise either renewed hair vigour, or even an end to baldness. (There is no cure for ordinary male baldness except castration, it must be emphasized.) The recipes have charm. 'Receipt to thicken hair and make it grow on a bald part' runs one. 'Take Roots of a Maiden Vine, Roots of Hemp, and Cores of soft Cabbages, of each two handfuls; dry and burn them; afterwards make a lye with the ashes. The head is to be washed with this lye three days successively, the part having been previously well rubbed with Honey.'

Or, more simply, 'Powder your head with powdered Parsley Seed at night, once in three or four months, and the hair will never fall off.'

Nettle juice was another specific. 'It is a good wash for the head, preventing the hair from falling and strengthening the roots. We used to keep a bowl of this mixed with a tablespoonful of vinegar on our toilet-tables and wash the roots of our hair with it about twice a month,' breathed an enthusiastic contributor to *The Girls Own Paper* of May 1894.

Rum was the basis of other remedies. Three onions placed in a quart of rum for twenty-four hours make up a lotion to rub on the bald scalp. 'The slightest odour of onions . . . evaporates in a few minutes.' Actually it doesn't. Nor does it improve the rum, if you decide to drink it.

Oddest of all was to find cantharides, or Spanish fly, in some of the old recipes for hair tonic. (Some link perhaps

45

between sexual performance and hair?) Morphet's American Hair Tonic contained two ounces of strong black tea, one gallon of boiling water, three ounces of glycerine, a whole quart of bay rum, and half an ounce of tincture of cantharides. Heaven forbid that the modern barber should start stocking this in addition to his other wares!

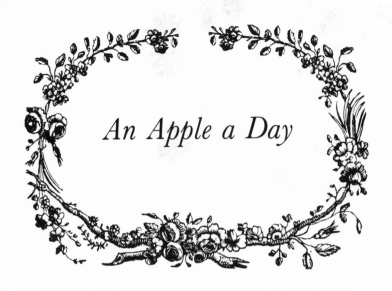

An Apple a Day

'THE BEST BEAUTIFYERS' said *The Lady's Newspaper* of the last century, 'are health, exercise and good temper.' And a thirteenth-century collection of physician's lore had this to say:

> For all brains the following things are hurtful; gluttony, drunkeness, late eating, much sleeping after food, tainted air, anger depressed spirits, much standing bare-headed, eating much or hastily, too much warmth, excessing watching, too much cold, curds, all kinds of nuts, frequent bathing, onions, garlic, yawning, smelling a white rose, excess of venery, too much music, singing and reading, strong drink before sleeping, restless sleep, too frequent fasting, wet feet.

Though one may not agree on all the details, the principles are clear. If you look after what you eat, what you do and how you feel, you will be not only healthier but also more beautiful. Our grandmothers were well aware of this. 'An apple a day keeps the doctor away' was one of their favourite sayings, and it is true that apples seem to agree with even the most delicate stomachs.

Orange juice, that trans-Atlantic breakfast staple, was not so much mentioned. But then oranges were exotic fruits. My mother remembers that the orange in the toe of her Christmas stocking was small, sweet, and blood red. Even the peel was highly prized. It was dried, and in her home used to be put on the drawing room fire to burn for its fragrance.

Not only fruits were valued as a source of health. Apart from anything else, by about January most of the apples carefully stored in sheds, attics or barns had gone wooly or bad. It was time to turn to other sources of health.

'Eat turnips and be beautiful' was an old saying. Turnip tops were also highly prized. At the end of the year when the root begins to go harsh and woody, the tops are at their best, I think.

Then there was succory (chicory to the modern gardener). The roots of these had been grown the year before, stored, and now could be grown blanched in the warmth of a kitchen cupboard. Culpeper maintained that chicory 'drives forth choleric and phlegmatic humours' and favourably affected 'swooning and passions of the heart'.

'Spinach and leeks bring lillies to the cheeks' was another old cottage saying. Spinach was available in summer, leeks in winter. Carrots were valued too, so much so that one beauty suggestion was a bowl of carrot soup for breakfast daily.

As summer arrived, delicious drinks were made up to promote internal health and external beauty. Lemonade was, of course, the most popular drink and I still think fresh lemonade takes a lot of beating. In winter I drink lemon, hot water, and honey. For a cold, add whisky. But in a hot summer there is nothing more refreshing than slightly weaker lemon and water, with ice and honey.

We seem today to have forgotten that other marvellous drink – the posset. John Nott of the Duke of Bolton's Kitchen, gives instructions for a French Posset.

Boil Three Pints of Cream, with some Nutmeg; sweeten a Pint of Wine in a Basin, set it over some Embers to warm a little; pour your Cream to it, sit it, and let it stand simmering over a Fire for an Hour and a half.

Scaled down a little, it sounds delicious.

At the other extreme are the herbal teas. From my garden I have picked peppermint, applemint, thyme, marjoram and pennyroyal, infused each in a little boiling water for a time, and drunk them with enjoyment. Wormwood is a little too bitter for me, and for some reason bergamot does not seem to grow very well with me. Some people add lemon juice, sugar, or honey to these herbal teas. Some recommend filling a huge jug with herbal tea and drinking it cold. Neither appeals to me, but I am sure that in any form they are a healthy addition to diet. (On somewhat the same lines, my husband's father used to drink the water in which green vegetables had been cooked – so as to avoid losing the 'goodness'.)

Since refrigerators were unknown in those early country days, our ancestors had to make far greater use of syrups and jams to preserve their fruit. Almost anything could be turned into jam, if wished. Culpeper certainly considered them an aid to health. 'This art' he says of conserving 'was plainly and first invented for delicacy, yet came afterwards to be of excellent use in physic. . . .'

As a rule-of-thumb cook, I use apple as a base for all my hedgerow jams. It makes life a great deal easier to have something you know will set, before you start adding ingredients of which you are less certain. When I am feeling most idle I just stew apples and blackberries – skins and all – and make apple-and-blackberry jam. By adding mixed spices, or cloves, or lemon juice, or even lemon peel, I can vary the flavour.

Dripping the mixture through an old lace curtain (as a jelly bag) before adding the sugar turns it into jelly. Using this system try adding elderberries instead of blackberries.

They give a better colour, though a less powerful flavour. In the same way sloes can be added for a deliciously tart plum-like jelly. I have tried hips too, but they did not seem to add a lot of flavour. Gerard, however, says that the fruit of the wild rose 'maketh most pleasant meats and banqueting dishes, as tarts and such like; the making whereof I commit to the cunning cooke, and teeth to eate them in the rich man's mouth.'

Then there is that other hedgerow delicacy – sloe gin. First buy your bottle of gin and pour off a quarter of it. Fill

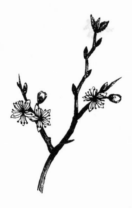

the empty space in the bottle with sloes, and add enough sugar to fill the cracks between the fruit. (Less, if you do not have a sweet tooth.) The difficult bit then is to leave it until Christmas, shaking the bottle only occasionally and admiring the rapidly growing redness of colour. For those who wonder what sloe gin has to do with beauty, I can only refer them to Culpeper.

The juice expressed from the unripe fruit is a very good remedy for fluxes of the bowels; it may be reduced by a gentle boiling to a solid consistence, in which state it will keep the year round.

Admittedly sloe gin includes alcohol, but then alcohol

lifts the spirits. And happiness is perhaps the best beauty aid of all. I have found no recipes for happiness. But in *The Compleat Houfewife* of 1744 I discovered something titled 'For a Distemper got by an ill Husband.'

> Take two pennyworth of gum-dragon, pick and clean it, and put it in an earthen pot; put to it as much red rose-water as it will drink up; stir it two or three times a day, till it is all dissolv'd into a jelly: then put in three grated nutmegs, and double-refin'd sugar to your taste, finely powder'd and a little cinnamon-water, no more than will leave it in a jelly; take the quantity of a nutmeg in the morning fasting, and last at night; but first prepare the body for it, by taking six pennyworth of pulvis sanctus in a posset-drink, and drink broth in the working.

It sounds a complicated remedy, but then the distemper got by an ill husband is a difficult disease to shift.

Sleep

INSOMNIA IS PERHAPS the most disagreeable bar to natural beauty. It corrodes the mind, wearies the frame, and depresses the spirits. We do not all need eight hours a day. There is an old saying about the hours of sleep, 'seven for a man, eight for a child, and nine for a fool.' But we do need sleep, real sleep. The sleep of sleeping drugs is a relief to the worried insomniac, but it is not a proper refreshment of the spirits. There is often a kind of pill hangover in the morning or else a hectic series of dreams, or otherwise dreamless sleep. But not being able to sleep is a fearful thing. In the long watches of the night minutes spread out into hours, or so it seems to the tormented mind. Sometimes the body develops odd tricks – pins and needles, palpitations of the heart, the throbbing of blood in the temples. At other times, an old anxiety surfaces into the mind and refuses to leave it.

There are the old remedies. Count sheep. Only for the non-mathematical such countings may be tedious. My own sheep leap one by one over a gate with increasingly mocking, deriding and sometimes monstrous faces. Count your blessings is another old saw. But the only thing the insomniac mind is likely to remember is its anxieties.

More useful was, I think, the household bedtime ritual of some three or four generations back. Some families still have this, but many simply turn off the television and go upstairs to bed.

Family prayers last thing at night were part of the old ritual. The Lord's Prayer was the most commonly included. Even the unbeliever must admit that the familiar words about daily bread, forgiveness for trespasses and avoidance of temptation may calm the mind. What is so odd is those people who happily accept and enjoy a morning routine – pottering, shaving, making-up etc – nevertheless avoid an evening one.

For some people a last minute drink is part of this ritual. Somebody once told me that Queen Victoria, influenced possibly by John Brown, her accompanying Scotsman, used to have a full bottle of whisky placed by her bed every night. The bottle was full because of her majestic status, not because she necessarily finished it. I have not checked this story for accuracy lest the harsh light of historical truth destroy it.

In any case, a last minute drink is not a bad idea. I have heard of an octogenerian lady who last thing at night drank a glass half full of port, half full of whisky. The most glamorous grandmother of them all, Barbara Cartland, recommends a last night-drink of hot water and honey. Many herbal enthusiasts swear by various herbal teas.

My own choice of herbal tea remedy for insomnia is passiflora. You can buy it in most good health food shops. I have it in dried form, and a tea made of the chopped-up leaves seems to bring on sleepiness without about twenty minutes. (Oddly enough, after that twenty minutes, the effect disappears.) But the taste, it must be admitted, is vile.

The most natural way to get a good night's sleep is to soothe and calm the mind. This means fixing it in some way so that it cannot wander back to the worries of daily life, or the fears for the future. Those who practise eastern religions or meditation have their own methods. But what of those who don't?

A poet friend of mine has an interesting mental trick. When he cannot sleep, he imagines he is walking towards a cave which is at the top of a hill. Inside the cave, there are many things that he particularly likes and values. He lets his mind dwell on these. As he peers into the cave, he makes a careful assessment of exactly what is there . . . and by this time he is sleeping.

I have tried this cave technique, but with no success. For me caves are too fear-producing, and my mind usually ends up by thinking of all the unpleasant things that are going to be inside the cave. But the principle of calming the mind by making it think of something pleasureable does seem to work. For me, the trick is to think of my garden. As I lie awake I plan exactly what I shall do in the future with various parts of the vegetable patch, and I refuse to think about the herbacious border which invariably needs weeding.

There are, of course, other small practical tricks. Always keep warm. Cold feet are a great hindrance to quick sleep. And if, for some reason, the mind refuses all diversion then I think it is better to turn on the light and read, or go and make a cup of tea, than to lie there in anxiety and sleepless torment. Some herbal writers suggest pillows of herbs to induce sleep, and hops are sold for this purpose. 'A bag to smell unto, or to cause one to sleep' in 1606 was made up of dried rose petals, powdered mint, and powdered cloves. 'Take that to bed with you and it will cause you to sleepe, and it is good to smell unto at other times.'

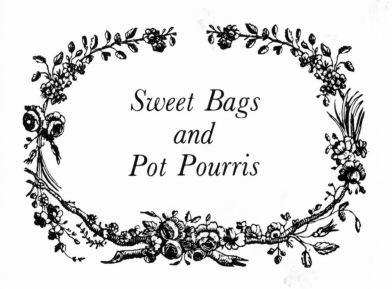

Sweet Bags
and
Pot Pourris

IT WAS NOT JUST the insomniac of a generation ago who valued a bag full of sweet smells. Sweet bags were made for all kinds of purposes – not least for the storing of clothes. Today only lavender bags seem to survive as a reminder of those earlier little bags. Lavender bags are indeed a pleasure, but it is quite unnecessarily unimaginative to confine such bags to just the one flower. *The Toilet of Flora* suggests:

> For this Purpose may be used different parts of the aromatic Plants; as Leaves of Southernwood, Dragon-wort, Balm, Mint, both garden and wild, Dittany, Ground-ivy, Bay, Hyssop, Lovage, Sweet Marjoram, Origanum, Pennyroyal, Thyme, Rosemary, Savory, Scordium, and Wild Thyme. The Flowers of the Orange, Lemon, Lime and Citron Tree, Saffron, Lavender, Roses, Lily of the Valley, Clove-july flower, Wallflower, Jonquil and Mace. Small green Oranges, Juniperberries, Nutmegs, and Cloves. Roots of Acorus, Bohemian Angelica, Oriental Costus, Sweet Flag, Orrice, Zedoary, etc. The Woods of Rhodium, Juniper, Caffia, St Lucia, Sanders etc. Gums, as Frankincense, Myrrh, Storax, Benjamin, Lab-

danum, Ambergrise and Amber. Barks as Canelia Alba,
Cinnamon etc.

It is an impressive total of suggestions, which gives a good
idea of the armoury of perfume available to the housewives
of an earlier age. Many of the ingredients we can no longer
buy. Others are only to be found, ageing and losing their
flavour, in supermarket rows of tiny pots. It is always better
to grow your own and dry them, than to buy the herbs ready
rubbed – both for cooking and for scenting.

I have two especial favourites. The first is southernwood,
also sometimes called lad's love. (I am told this is a reference
not to the amorous nature of young men, but a corruption of
Our Lady's Love.) It has a weird scent, not entirely
pleasing, and some say a sprig should be included in every
nosegay to remind one that among life's sweets are also its
bitters. It has the reputation, perhaps because of this smell,
of keeping away moths. Moths, or not, I just like its odd
pungent smell among my sweaters. Sometimes I add some
wormwood, an even more bitter smelling herb with lovely
grey foliage. Or I make up a separate wormwood bag.

My other favourite sweet bag could not be more different.
It is made of scented geranium leaves. These come from
special geraniums – not those boringly repeated park
flowers, their red foliage harsh against the tired grass, their
leaves smelling faintly but uninterestingly. The scented
geraniums have romantic names. There is the Prince of
Orange with appropriately orangey leaves, Mabel Grey
with curiously deep cut leaves and a strong citrus smell, Joy
Lucille (pepperminty), Clorinda (cedar-scented) and then
the incomparable common Attar of Roses. The most
common variety is called Graveolens, a name which does
no justice to its delicious scent. Nearly all of the scented
varieties will make marvellous sweet bags, and I have found
that mine last for about two years. The bags are simple to
make – just fill them with the dried rubbed leaves. If a bag
seems to lose its savour give it another rub or two. Scented

geraniums are delicious in other ways – in jams, jellies, stewed fruit, in baths and, of course *pot-pourris*.

The art of the *pot-pourri* is another neglected Victorian piece of housewifery. In principle, there are two sorts of *pot-pourri* – wet and dry. If you are content with a very simple, rather fugitive *pot-pourri* you can simply dry the leaves of aromatic herbs (not forgetting scented geraniums) and add lots of rose leaves. A few unscented but gaily coloured leaves or petals will add to the visual beauty. But to get the full virtue of a *pot-pourri*, something more must be added. Not the fixative oils that are poured over bought *pot-pourris*, but a strengthener like orris root powder.

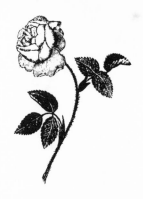

I am indebted to the Nicholls family who lived in Honiton, Devon, around the year 1870, for my *pot-pourri* recipe. It was a family which included thrifty wives, ladies' maids and maiden aunts. Many were the family recipe books in which herbal remedies and other bits of housewifery were written down. Their recipe for West of England *pot-pourri* was as follows:

Pick the flowers as early as possible as soon as the dew is off the blooms. Red flowers are better than white or paler colours. Gather petals from about thirty-six blooms and dry them in an airing cupboard.

Take a large china jar and press down in it alternate layers of petals and bay salts. After a week, give the lot a vigorous stir with a knitting needle.

Then add the following – two ounces of orris root, a few tonquin beans, and crushed cinnamon sticks. Also one teaspoonful of allspice. Stick cloves into an orange, dry in the oven, and add to the *pot-pourri*.

Dry a handful of sage leaves and rosemary, a sprig of thyme,

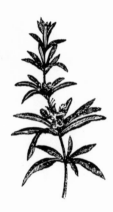

a few scented geranium leaves (crushed), some sweet woodruff and stir into the mixture. Use freely in drawers or in muslin bags. It is also excellent when placed in a small china bowl in a bedroom.

From this you will no doubt deduce that the original china pot was a large one. Family tradition has it that the Nicholls used an old china jerry.

Finally a recipe for an even older form of scenting the air – 'burning perfume'.

Take a quarter of pound of damask-rose leaves, beat them by themselves, an ounce of orrice-root sliced very thin and steep'd in rose-water, beat them well together, and put to it two grains of musk, as much civet, two ounces of Benjamin finely powder'd; mix all together and add a little powder'd sugar, and make them up into little round cakes, and lay them singly on papers to dry; set them in a window where the sun comes, they will dry in two or three days: make them in July.

That was from *The Compleat Houfewife* of 1744. Those who may wonder if the labour of burning perfumes, making Hungary Water, sweet bags, *Huile Antique de la Rose* and other suggestions in this book are worthwhile should perhaps think over the opening words of *The Toilet of Flora*.

The same Share of Grace and Attractions is not possessed by all of them but while the Improvement of their Persons is the indispensable Duty of those who have been little favoured by Nature, it should not be neglected even by the few who have received the largest portion of her Gifts. The same Art which will communicate to the former the Power of pleasing, will enable the latter to extend the Empire of their Beauty.

Suppliers

IT IS SOMETIMES difficult to buy all the pharmaceutical and herbal ingredients that you need to make your own cosmetics. The following firms can usually help.

John Bell and Croyden, 50–54 Wigmore St, London W1 (Telephone number 01-935 5555) stocks many of the vital ingredients such as beeswax, emulsifying wax B.P. etc. It has a postal department.

Culpeper, herbalists, 21 Bruton St, London W1 stock orris root and other herbal products.

J. and B. Hugo, Ashfields Herb Nursery, Hinstock, Market Drayton, Salop (Telephone number Sambrook 392) will supply healthy herb plants and seeds. Send 25p for their informative catalogue.

Index